Little
Indulgences

NANNA

Little Indulgences

More Than 400 Ways to Be Good to Yourself

Cynthia MacGregor

CONARI PRESS

First published in 2003 by Conari Press,
an imprint of Red Wheel/Weiser, LLC
York Beach, ME
With offices at:
368 Congress Street
Boston, MA 02210
www.redwheelweiser.com

LIBRARY OF CONGRESS CATALOGING-IN-PUBLICATION DATA
MacGregor, Cynthia.
  Little indulgences : more than 400 ways to be good to yourself / Cynthia MacGregor.
    p. cm.
Includes bibliographical references and index.
  ISBN 1-57324-873-8
  1. Conduct of life--Miscellanea. 2. Quality of life--Miscellanea. I. Title.
  BF637.C5M32 2003
  646.7--dc21

                       2003008484

Typeset in Deepdene by Kathleen Wilson Fivel
Cover design by David A. Freedman
Printed in Canada.
TCP

10 09 08 07 06 05 04 03
 8 7 6 5 4 3 2 1

Acknowledgments

In alphabetical order, thanks to:
Andrew Brownlee, Cindy Crawford (not the famous one), Norm Edelman, Lars Hanson, Andrea Kalina, Jesse Leaf, Bob Lebensold, Bess Metcalf, Lori Paige, Mari-Jean Phillips, Zac Phillips, Ken Pinkham, Jennifer Radalin, Bruce Wallace, and Ruth Wenig.

Indulge Yourself Today

Today is a special day.

Okay, so maybe it's not your birthday. Or the anniversary of your wedding (or divorce). Or the day you start your dream job. Or your child's birthday. Or a national holiday. Or any other milestone.

But why can't it be a special day anyhow?

Any day can be a special day if you want it to be. You give special treats to the other people who are important to you. You buy them little gifts or cook them special foods. But aren't *you* important too? Certainly you deserve special treatment sometimes.

The treat you give yourself doesn't have to be an all-day thing (although it could be). Sometimes just a quick pick-me-up, ten minutes spent doing something special, something meaningful, something nice for yourself is all you need to turn an ordinary day, or even a "down" day, into a special day. Just to give you a heads-up, I've marked some of these with the little clock for *Instant Indulgences*. I recommend you pick one and do it right away.

Sometimes, we all need a special day. Sometimes it's to help us get over the blues. Sometimes it's to help us get over the blahs. Sometimes it's because we're in a celebratory mood and need an occasion to celebrate. Sometimes it's because we *have* an occasion to celebrate and need a way to do it. And sometimes it's "just because."

Whatever your reason (although you don't *have* to have one at all), if you need or want a special day, there are plenty of ways to give yourself one. Ways that are extravagant, ways that are budget-priced, ways that are completely cost-free. Things you can do alone or with a friend, at home or away, quietly or exuberantly. I've indicated these with the calendar page for *All Day Indulgences*. Mark your calendar now. When can you devote a whole day to yourself? Choose an all-dayer and make a date with yourself.

 Some of the indulgences in this book are the *Reward Over Time* kind. Begin an exercise program today and you'll reap benefits— some now and some over time. Ditto starting a more healthy diet. Or beginning to keep a journal.

 And then there are those times when the best thing you can do for yourself is to do something for someone else. These I call *Generous Indulgences*.

This book is filled with indulgences—treats and activities for every taste and budget. Open it up at random when you're feeling down. Use it as a planning tool. That's right, you should actually *plan* to be good to yourself. Keep it handy for that inevitable day when you want to treat yourself but you're feeling so blue or bored or tired that you're fresh out of inspiration.

Feel free to improvise. Start a list of your own indulgences. But, whatever you do, be good to yourself. Today can be *your* special day. (And so can tomorrow, if you want.)

Throw yourself a half-birthday party.

Call an old friend you haven't talked to in ages,
catch up, and yak at length.

Write a poem about someone you love—
your beloved, a close friend, a family member.
As you write it, you'll remember
all the things you love about that person,
and why he or she is so special to you.

Buy yourself
an extravagant bouquet.

Exercise.
Do your regular exercise routine or start a new one.
Rent or borrow exercise tapes, go for a walk,
learn yoga, play golf, do some sit-ups,
or just run up and down the stairs ten times.

❧

Have your legs waxed.

❧

Treat yourself to a session at a tanning salon,
or buy a nice self-tanning product (safer!)—
especially if you have the midwinter blahs.

Volunteer your time to the local headquarters
of your preferred political party or, if it's
election time, the headquarters of your
favorite candidate (local or national).
Knowing that you're making a difference
in how the government is run will make
a difference in how you feel about yourself.

ॐ

Have your car washed, waxed, and detailed.

Send flowers to the local nursing home——it will make you feel fabulous.

Go away for the weekend.
You don't have to go far,
and it doesn't have to be expensive.
Visit someone special, or stay at a quaint inn.
Bring a friend or go alone.
What you need is a change of scene, a change of pace.

Buy yourself a bunch of helium balloons
and turn them loose all over your house.
Have a little fun and bat one around.
Then walk through the park and
give them away to passersby.

Cook a new food—one you've
never even attempted before.
It doesn't have to be as exotic as alligator meat,
buffalo steaks, or chocolate-covered ants.
It could be beef or chicken cooked
in a sauce you've never dared to try.

Learn a new computer skill or program.

Learn to belly dance.

Mark a memory. Sit at the computer or curl up with a notepad and a good pen and remember—in exquisite detail—one of the most wonderful things that's ever happened to you. It could be your first kiss, your wedding day, a surprise birthday party that truly was a surprise. Dwell on how wonderful you felt then and feel those emotions returning now.

Get all of your jewelry professionally cleaned.

Plant something special in your yard—
a fruit tree, a fragrant bush that blossoms in your
favorite color, or some brightly cheerful flowers.
Think of the pleasures you'll have from it
in the years to come—and how it will
improve your property's looks and value.

Decide you're going to learn to play an instrument
(*another* instrument if you play one already).
Buy an inexpensive electronic musical keyboard
(the kind that simulates any instrument) or rent an
electric guitar or even a harp. It's never too late.

Infuse the air in your home with
a sweet scent—spray a *cool* light bulb
with perfume, turn on the light,
and let the warmth of the bulb
spread the scent through the air.

Smell a tomato plant.

Inhale deeply.

Again.

Again.

Buy all new bras and panties!

Rent or borrow a convertible on a day when you have a lot of local errands to do or wish to visit a friend who lives an hour away. Put the top down, of course!

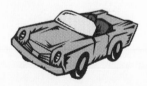

Make a cave, or a fort, or a play house.
Drape a sheet over a table.
Put down some pillows.
Crawl in with a good book.
Or a snack.
Or your favorite stuffed animal.
(If your kids are nice to you, you *might* let them in!)

Have your initials painted
on your car in elegant, large letters.

Go to a salon and have your eyebrows
professionally shaped.

Host a Recipe-Exchange Party

Tired of cooking the same old dishes? You don't need to buy a whole new cookbook. Call up a group of friends and organize a recipe exchange! Since you're the hostess, you can specify that each guest bring only main courses, or only desserts, or only "sides," or only chicken recipes—or you can ask each guest to bring recipes enough for a complete meal. Let your guests know how many will be coming and ask them to make that many copies of each of the recipes they're bringing. You could even make the get-together a potluck, with each guest bringing one of the dishes for which she's contributing a recipe.

*Put your spare change in other
people's expired parking meters.
You will smile knowing that in a small
way you are someone's guardian angel.*

Get your bellybutton pierced,
if that's appealing to you.

Start a gratitude notebook.
(A small, inexpensive notebook you can carry in
your bag works just as well as a fancy journal.)
List all the things you are grateful for.
Add to your notebook from time to time.
And read it over when you feel like
life is dealing you a nasty hand.

Rearrange the furniture in one of the rooms
of your house. Make the room more practical,
workable, or more aesthetically pleasing, or just
highlight a piece of furniture you're proud of.

Suit yourself.

Please yourself.

Have fun.

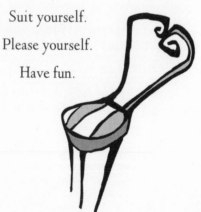

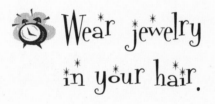

Wear jewelry
in your hair.

Hire a limousine to drive you
and someone special to dinner.

See if you can still play the ball-bouncing games
of your childhood, like "A, My Name Is Alice."
If you don't have a Spaldeen (pink rubber ball),
a tennis ball will do just as well.

Read some young adult fiction,
such as Nancy Drew or Harry Potter.

Give yourself permission to procrastinate.

Learn how to make candy at home.

Go vintage-clothing shopping.
Buy a fabulous trench coat or fancy dress.

List all the ways you are a nice (or interesting, or smart, or loyal) person. Now, record this list in your own voice and keep the tape on hand to play back whenever you need that reminder.

Write down the details of your favorite childhood toy to preserve the memory for your kids or grandkids (even if you don't have any of either yet).

Work up a clown routine
and experiment with suitable
clothes and makeup.
Now you can entertain at parties,
volunteer to visit hospitalized kids,
cheer up the residents at nursing
homes, and bring happiness
wherever you go in your
costume—whether it's
a do-good effort,
a paid performance,
or just for fun.

Buy a single carnation (or rose, or other flower)
and place it in a bud vase in the center of your
dining room table (or in some other location
in your home where you'll see it often).

Start a house-decorating scrapbook—
cut out pictures from magazines that inspire you
and fantasize about your perfect home.

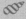

Wash your hair, and take the time to give yourself a
thorough scalp massage while you wash it. Better yet,
get a friend to do it for you.

Go out in the backyard and throw a Frisbee.

⚭

Buy yourself some *expensive* chocolates
from an upscale candy shop—where
you can pick exactly what you want.
(No more, "Ugh . . . raspberry!"
when you're looking for butter cream!)

Throw a tea party and ask each person to bring
two of their favorite herbs or spices.
Then have everyone create exotic, new tea blends
from all the different ingredients offered.

Do an Internet search to find
a childhood friend you've lost touch with.

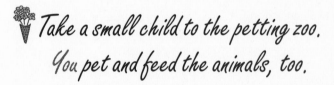

Take a small child to the petting zoo.
You pet and feed the animals, too.

Write down or record the story of a pet you had
as a child. If you didn't have a real pet, did you
have an imaginary one? If you didn't have an
imaginary one then, would you like one now?

❧

*Buy yourself half a dozen plants for your house,
including at least a couple of plants that
flower or have colorful leaves.*

This morning, fix your hair and makeup extra-nice, as if you were going out somewhere special, even though it's just an ordinary day. Now, take a good, long look at yourself in the mirror. It doesn't feel like just an ordinary day anymore, does it?

❧

Hire a window-washer
and get your windows sparkling.

Set aside a Sunday morning to cook and freeze a week's worth of dinners. (Choose recipes for foods that freeze well.) Now you'll have a "night off" from cooking every day for the next week—or for any seven days, not necessarily consecutive, that you choose.

Rent a horse from a local stable for an hour's trail ride.

Give some time to a charitable or other do-good effort. Be a "Big Sister," teach an adult to read, or simply stuff envelopes for a fund-raising drive for the local library or homeless shelter. By doing good for others, you'll feel great about yourself!

Start an herb-garden outdoors
or on your windowsill.

Deep condition your hair.

Your Mysterious Admirer

If you're single, order a bouquet of flowers sent to yourself at work—or even one bouquet every other day for a week. When your co-workers ask who the bouquet was from, you can answer (in all honesty), "There was no card." Let them wonder who cares about you enough to send you flowers. Let them speculate on your Mysterious Admirer. Let them see you in a whole new light.

Dig out your old photo albums and just reminisce
alone, with your special someone,
with your mom, or with your best friend.

Buy a big, floppy men's shirt to wear yourself.

Go to a karaoke bar and sing!

If you don't have a regular cleaning person,
hire a housecleaning service to come in
and thoroughly clean your home.

After washing your hair, dry it in the sunshine.

Host a Christmas-in-July party. Get folks to bring gifts for homeless children.

Write yourself coupons for special treats—
a shopping spree, a milkshake, a new blouse.

Take singing lessons.

Plant some tomatoes, or some other fruit or veggie,
in your garden. Enjoy the connection with a growing
thing now as you work at tending your crop, enjoy
the fruits of your labors later as you harvest your
produce, and then enjoy your bounty at the table.

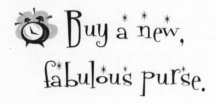

Buy a new, fabulous purse.

Make a list of three things—just three—that you honestly believe you *could* (not *should* but *could*) improve about yourself. These could be physical, emotional, or situational. Now write down two steps you could take toward attaining each of these three goals. Congratulate yourself on your resolve to start right away. (Don't you feel better about yourself already?)

Locate a perfumery that makes fragrances to order
and have them create a scent especially for you.

Have your upholstered furniture
professionally cleaned.

Visit a travel agency and load up on brochures for two
vacations: one you reasonably believe you can take
sometime within the next year (even if it's just a car
trip to a neighboring state), and one you can't possibly
afford but can have a grand time daydreaming about.

Start a "yard improvement" notebook. Plan things showy and spectacular—perhaps a trellis or arbor, an elaborate bird feeder, a gazebo, a porch-type swing, a bright flowerbed, a koi pond.

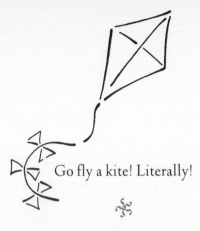

Go fly a kite! Literally!

❊

Call up whoever the baker in your family is—
your mom or sister, aunt or cousin,
or maybe it's even one of the guys—
and get the recipe for her (or his!) signature dessert.
Try to duplicate it, and eat as much as you want.

Get a bonsai tree and prune it
in deliciously wonderful ways.

Buy yourself a telescope and get to know more about
the kind of stars that don't get written about in the
gossip columns—the ones that twinkle, twinkle.

Remember all the good things
your parents have done for you over the years.

Take Ten with a Tree

Spend ten relaxing minutes in quiet contemplation of a tree. Observe the overall shape of the whole tree—is it symmetrical, does it resemble anything else, is it pleasing to the eye? Commit to memory the shape of the individual leaves—have you ever really studied the shape of an individual oak, elm, or maple leaf before?

Observe the bark—is it rough, relatively smooth, craggy; does it resemble alligator skin, parchment, or some other object or texture? What about the ground beneath the tree—how does the part of the earth that is shaded by the tree differ from the area surrounding it—is the grass there thinner, sparser, shorter; are any other forms of vegetation present or absent that are different from what's found in the area outside the tree's shade? Now, lie down under the tree and stare up at the branches. Feel peace steal over you.

Read the employment ads—and not just the ones
pertaining to your current career, but *every* ad.
Imagine yourself changing careers in midstream.
What else would you *like* to do?
Now, are any of these temptations actually feasible?

Splurge on a day at a spa.

Visit a winery and participate
in a wine-tasting session.

Declare a Sunday for yourself on a Wednesday—or any other weekday. Take a personal day off from work and enjoy a day of indolence— or a day crammed with as many pleasurable activities as can fit into eight hours of playing hooky.

Buy yourself a few bags of fancy, expensive coffees.

Spend an afternoon going over your
school yearbooks, camp yearbooks,
or scrapbooks of childhood souvenirs.

Go to a meadow and pick an armful of wildflowers.
Never mind if some of them are
actually weeds—as long as they appeal to you!

✤

Dream up a recipe it would be fun to cook
and/or to eat. It might be a lavish main course,
a new hors d'oeuvre, or simply a new variation on
chicken salad. For now, just write it down, but do
plan to treat yourself by actually trying it soon.

∞

Buy some attractive stepping stones for your garden.

*Contribute to a charity
that's meaningful to you—
even if $5 or $10 is all
you can afford to give right now.*

Take an early morning sun bath,
while the sun is strong enough
only to kiss you with its warmth,
not make you sweat or burn.

Trim your bangs.

Go to the department store fragrance counter
and try on some new and different perfumes.
Try the men's cologne department, too—
you never know what you might find!

❧

Buy yourself some caviar or smoked oysters
and indulge yourself with the finer things in life.

Take a long, hot soak in the tub by candlelight.

Subscribe to a new and exciting magazine.

Place inspirational quotations
throughout your home—
on the refrigerator,
over the fireplace,
next to the bathtub.

Plan a party. Maybe an intimate lunch with two close
friends or a big, all-out blowout for a near-future
Saturday night. Don't just write down the date or
form the intention. Actually begin planning.

Buy a dozen new pairs of socks you don't
really need. Get your favorite kind, be it
trouser socks, tube socks, or fuzzy slipper socks,
or buy some in wild colors just for fun.

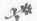

Have those old family movies transferred
to videotape, and plan to spend an evening
(or several) watching them.

Install soft-colored light bulbs in some or all of your
lamps and lighting fixtures, then turn them on and
see what a difference the hues make in your house.

*Treat yourself to extravagant,
striking accessories for your bathroom.*

Nature's Lullaby

Dig out from the closet (or borrow) a sleeping bag, or make up a bedroll, and sleep out on your screened-in terrace, back porch, or similar protected-but-outdoorsy projection from your house. Listen to the night sounds as you drift off, and really listen to the birdcalls as the day breaks. (What else do you hear? Frogs? Crickets? A train in the distance? Isn't it wonderful how different the sounds are under these circumstances?)

Read the restaurant reviews
in your local paper or magazine.
Pick up the phone and make that reservation.
Go and enjoy!

*Make yourself a fruit smoothie—
it's refreshing, healthful, and colorful!*

Write a fan letter to your favorite singer,
actress, writer, or other performer or artist.
Don't gush—say *why* you're a fan,
praising the person's work honestly.
Who knows—you might get a personal reply.

Consider getting a tattoo.
Think about what designs or words you
would like permanently attached to your skin.
If you can't commit to a permanent tattoo,
try a henna tattoo—they're just as striking,
last for weeks, and don't hurt a bit!

Lady, go buy a new pair of shoes!

Shop for new body oils.

Buy some old wooden furniture from a garage sale,
yard sale, or flea market. Have fun painting it a bold
color, or refinishing it to match your décor.

Chew some bubble gum and attempt
to blow the world's largest, most perfect bubble.

If you have a CD burner, make mixed-music
CDs for your friends and mail them
as a surprise—it will make you feel great!

Relax in a hammock, swinging gently back and forth.
Bring a good book and/or some music with you—or just
lie there observing nature with your eyes, nose, and ears.

The next time you visit your favorite restaurant,
don't order your favorite food.
Order something new and different and daring!

If you're usually surrounded by people, spend a day all by yourself and enjoy the solitude—and the deliciousness—of your own company.

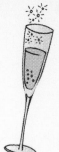

Have a glass of champagne after dinner.

If you have a few dollars to spare
(and you don't have a gambling problem!)
a trip to the horse track, dog track, or a
nearby casino may be just the pick-me-up
you want—whether or not you win.
But who knows . . . ?

Try on hats.

Turn some beach-combing treasures into jewelry.

Using chocolate syrup, club soda, milk,
and ice cream, make yourself an old-fashioned ice
cream soda. (Don't worry about the calories.
As long as cholesterol or sugar isn't a major health
issue with you, you can cheat this once!)

Give yourself permission to sit down (right now!)
and simply daydream (for at least fifteen minutes).

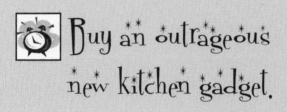 Buy an outrageous new kitchen gadget.

Saturate a rag with vanilla extract and run
it through the dryer to make your house smell great.

Pay a professional organizer to bring order
to the chaos of your closets.

*Spend an afternoon at the museum of your choice
all by yourself, so you can move at your own pace.*

Test drive that new car you've been wanting—even
if you know you can't afford to buy it right now.
If you love the car, the drive will be fun.
And if you find you *don't* love it, you'll feel
better about not being able to afford it.

۶

Buy a deck of tarot cards and do readings for yourself.

Start a recipe chain letter. The person receiving the letter has to send a recipe to the top name on the list, cross that name off, insert her name at the bottom, and send the list on to four other people.

Light some incense and practice meditating.

જી

Go to the lake, river, or ocean
and watch the boats go by.
Wave.

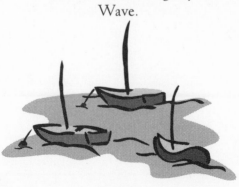

If you've never liked your first name, pick a new one!
You can legally change it, or you can just spread the
word to your friends, "From now on, please call me
Gwendolyn." You can even send formal or whimsical
announcements of your name change.

*Buy a pair of false eyelashes
and don't wait for New Year's to wear them!*

Make a sundial in your backyard.

Write a letter to your congressman or other suitable politician, sounding off about something that's bothering you and is within the government's ability to change. Your actions just might make your corner of the world a little better place to live, and in any case, you'll feel better for at least having taken a step to try to make it happen.

Spend fifteen minutes or several hours playing with a child. Let yourself go. Whether you're playing horsie with a two-year-old, climbing a tree with a six-year-old, or playing hide 'n' go seek with a ten-year-old, you'll not only give the child a good time, you'll get in touch with your own inner child.

Make a wonderful chicken stock
and your whole house will smell marvelous.

Decide now to approach your
next birthday as if you were a kid.
Decide what games you're going to play
(pin the tail, bobbing for apples,
charades, relay races).
Buy noisemakers,
party hats, and balloons.
Make the party
a festive return to childhood
for you and your guests.

Buy a new cookbook.

Gather a bunch
of old family photographs
and create a collage
to hang in your home.

Step out of your wardrobe comfort zone
and try something completely different.
Are you a trendy dresser?
Why not try a suit today.
Are you conservative?
Wear feathers in your hair.
You might just learn something about yourself.

Buy music from an international location you've
always wanted to visit—Greece, Africa, Russia.

Visit a gourmet and/or ethnic food emporium.

Go to a flower show.

Borrow a book-on-tape from the library
to listen to during your morning commute.

Take cuttings from your houseplants and repot them (or put them in water to grow roots—whichever is appropriate to the type of plant). Think of all the new greenery you'll have growing in your house soon!

Get Lasik treatments for your eyes
and throw away your glasses!

Borrow your child's basketball,
go out in the driveway, and shoot some
hoops—even if you last tried to sink a
ball in a basket in the gym in junior high.

Set your alarm clock, program your coffee maker,
get up early—and head out to watch the sun rise.

Take a class in flower-arranging or napkin-folding.

Pack a basket with some special treats (homemade
or store-bought) and picnic in a nearby park.
Do it even if you live in the city.
Do it even if you work nine-to-five.
Ask a friend to share if you like.

❧

Build a sandcastle.

Call up your mom and dad
and tell them how much
you love them and why.
Share the happiest memories
of your childhood.
Knowing how good you're
making them feel will give
you a good feeling, too.

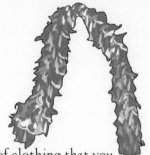

Buy an article of clothing that you
really don't need but looks divine on you.

If there is helicopter sightseeing available
in your area, treat yourself to a ride.

Set up an inflatable wading pool in the backyard,
get into a bathing suit, and frolic
and splash like a four-year-old!

⌇

Buy yourself a particularly pretty, large,
special, fantastic coffee mug. You may also
enjoy drinking soups, other beverages, or
even lunchtime stews from your new mug.

ⓖ

Make a journal or scrapbook.

⌇

Try a new variety of wine or flavor of ice cream.

Create a video diary.
Ask your friends to talk
into the camera about the current
topics of the day and edit the
snippets into a commentary
on the times you are living in.
Tuck it away for posterity.

Arrange with a friend to leave your kids with her while you go do all your errands unencumbered.

Wear a flower in your hair.

The next time you make popcorn, simmer some hot chocolate to go with it. Be decadent—add three marshmallows (or a *huge* dollop of whipped cream) and one splash of vanilla extract.

Buy yourself an old-fashioned clock. A clock that ticks. A clock that either chimes or cuckoos on the hour and the half-hour. A clock with character that's fun to listen to and interesting to look at.

Notable Notepads

Make personalized stationery. Using your computer scanner, scan in a good (or funny!) picture of yourself and paste it onto a file with "From the desk of" or "From the fevered brain of" or "From the cluttered desk of" or some other suitable line, either serious or funny. You now have the option of using this as a template and running it out straight from your computer, typing memos and letters on it, or printing out one good copy and having a commercial printer print 100 or 500 copies, which you can then handwrite memos on if you wish.

Buy all new makeup in new shades:
lipstick, nail polish, eye shadow, mascara, blush!

Adopt a parrot and teach it how to speak.

Turn up your car radio
and sing at the top of your lungs.

Use different oils on your salad—sesame, mushroom,
walnut—visit a co-op for even more ideas.

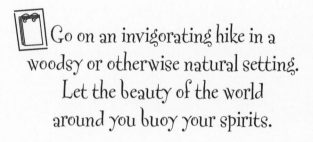 Go on an invigorating hike in a woodsy or otherwise natural setting. Let the beauty of the world around you buoy your spirits.

Set up an aquarium and fill it with tropical fish.
Get to know each one personally!

Have an enlargement made of your favorite
of all the photos you've ever taken, frame it,
and hang it on your home or office walls.

Tonight, make your absolutely all-time favorite
recipe for dinner. Why not serve dinner
on your *good* china on a beautiful tablecloth?
Light candles—even if you're eating alone!

Pajama Party!

Host an old-fashioned sleepover party for a few friends. You'll get pleasure twice—once now, as you plan the party, and then again later, when you actually have it. Every guest needs to bring her own sleeping bag or bedroll, and you'll all sleep on the living room floor. So what if you're not eight or even eighteen anymore? Twenty-eight-year-olds and even people much older—if they're limber enough and haven't lost their joy of childhood fun—can enjoy getting together for an evening that starts out perhaps with dinner (order pizzas!), continues with popping popcorn and roasting marshmallows (got a fireplace? a backyard barbecue grill? a can of Sterno?), might include playing boxed games or renting a movie, and definitely ought to include telling ghost stories, sharing "My Most Embarrassing Moment," and perhaps playing Truth or Dare.

Take a walk on your lunch hour.

Place a bouquet of fragrant flowers on your
night table. Enjoy the sight of the bouquet
gracing your bedroom, and as you drift off or
wake up, you'll smell that wonderful fragrance
for as many days as the flowers last.

Buy a pair of contact lenses that changes your eye
color—even if you don't need prescription lenses.

Don't play the stereo or TV in the house or in your car for an entire day. Cut out the background noise and instead, just listen to the world around you.

Ask for a dinner invitation from a friend
who's both a good cook and good company.

Write a children's book—who knows?
Maybe it'll be published!

Float a single fragrant flower in an elegant soup
tureen in the center of your coffee table.

*Go see a live show—a night at the theatre, the ballet,
or a concert. Go alone or with someone special.*

Make a snow angel,
even if you're on a sandy beach.

Investigate the Peace Corps.
Even if you don't think you'd ever join,
it's fun to imagine helping
people in far-off places.

Order a new welcome mat with your name on it.

Consider having permanent eyeliner
and/or blush tattooed onto you.

If someone has been good to you in the course of doing his or her job—such as a worker at a local store, the receptionist in your dentist's office, or someone in an office you do business with—write to his or her employer and let them know. Again, you'll feel almost as good after writing that letter as the person you're writing about will feel after his or her boss reads it.

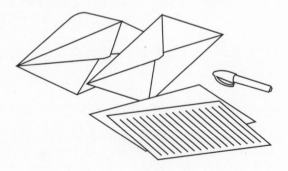

Learn to tango.

Spray some real cloth handkerchiefs
with your favorite perfume. Put one
in your bag and the others into a drawer.

Go to bed early and catch up on that
much-needed sleep you've been missing.

Go for a walk in the moonlight, away from street
lights, and enjoy the panoply of stars above. Watch
carefully—you might be lucky and get to see a meteor!

Skip rope down your street.

When you have the house to yourself,
blast your favorite music as loud as you care to play it.

Write a short, inspirational poem (or just a sentence) in lipstick on your bathroom mirror.

Buy a new day planner or a personal digital assistant (PDA) and spend the afternoon transferring all your appointments and addresses to your new organizer.

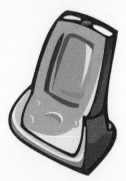

Comfort foods tend to be warm, simple, and associated with our childhood. They're the foods many people turn to when they're feeling sick or when they need an emotional pick-me-up. But you don't need to be sick to turn to comfort foods. What's wrong with a little comfort any time you want to be good to yourself?

Write a note (or list) addressed to your best friend on the topic of "Why You're My Best Friend," and ask her to write something similar addressed to you. Now exchange notes/lists and read what she has to say about you while enjoying knowing the pleasure she's getting out of your note or list.

Got wrinkles, spider veins, crows' feet, or something
else about your appearance bothering you?
Consult a doctor—maybe there's
a simple and affordable treatment.

❧

Buy yourself a book of crossword puzzles, or a jigsaw
puzzle, and lose yourself for an hour in puzzle-solving.

❧

Rent a movie you might otherwise overlook—
a foreign film with subtitles, an old silent movie,
a martial arts action flick.

Hold a yard sale,
clearing out all the stuff
that you really don't need
and that is taking up space,
and make a profit on your clean-up.

Visit a playground.
Just watch and listen to the kids.
Swing on the swings.

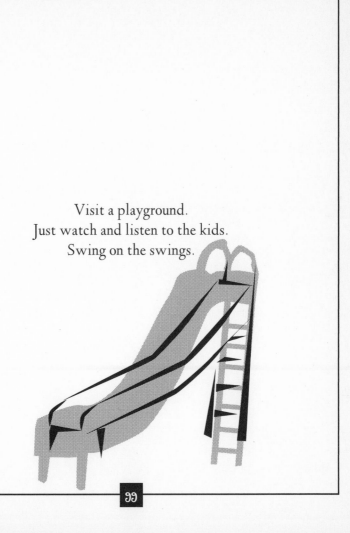

Drag out the old home movies, pop some popcorn, and have a real family home movie night. (If you live alone, you can still enjoy whatever family home movies you have on hand.)

Write a letter-to-the-editor of your local paper and get something off your chest. (There ... don't you feel better now?)

L ie in the backyard for half an hour of just listening to the birdsong, observing the squirrels, daydreaming, and not doing anything overtly productive. (I say "overtly" because you may find that, while your mind is cleared of its usual concerns, some wonderful ideas come to you.) If you're a sun-worshipper, bask in the sun as you lie there; if you're sun-shy (concerned about burning or skin safety), you can always do your stretching-out in the shade.

Browse through a seed or plant catalog.

Go to a mall recording studio
and record yourself singing your favorite song.

Sign up for an evening course.
It might be something practical,
something purely fun,
or something you've always
wanted to learn.

Visit an apple orchard
and pick your own bushels.
Make a pie.

Buy a pint of your favorite ice cream
and eat the whole thing at one sitting.

Have your teeth professionally whitened.

Go to a fashion show and sit in the front row.
Bring a notebook and make people
wonder just who you are.

Visit a relative's or friend's grave.
Not a *happy* thing to do, but one that may
bring you peace—and remind you of good times, too.

Buy a pair of silk pajamas or a sexy nightie.

*Invite someone special
to join you and splurge
on a special meal
in a good restaurant.*

Make a paper airplane and sail it around the room.

Light a fire in the fireplace—or crank up the air
conditioner—and curl up on the sofa with a cup
of tea and a letter you've saved, perhaps for years,
that's worth rereading. (It need not be a love letter;
it might be an "I appreciate you" note from your best
friend, the first letter your child ever sent home
from camp, or some other special treasure of saved
correspondence.)

Make a list:
Write down all the reasons your friends like you
and all the things you like about yourself.
Mail the list to yourself.

If you're not accustomed to taking daily naps,
take one for the sheer decadence of borrowing time
from the middle of your busy day for self-indulgence.

Make a list of how you'd spend the lottery jackpot
if you won it. Go out and buy a ticket,
even if you never buy one normally.
If you usually buy one, buy an extra one.
See—you've just doubled your chances of winning!

Plan to visit your old college
during homecoming week.

*Get your child's finger-paints out
and have a wonderfully messy time.*

Buy marshmallow fluff, butterscotch topping,
hot fudge, whipped cream, maraschino cherries,
crushed nuts, and your *two* favorite flavors
of ice cream. Construct a splendiferous sundae,
and have a ball eating it. (Oops ... I left out the
sprinkles ... but you don't have to!)

Start a vacation club bank account.

Weed out the clothing you no longer wear—
think charity donation, unless you have
a same-sized friend you prefer to offer the clothes to.

Bring your pets to be groomed—imagine how nice it
will be to have them around when they smell clean.

Go see the circus.

Buy a beautiful journal
to hold your most secret thoughts.

Forgive someone.
Decide for yourself whether or not
to tell the person you've forgiven.
Sometimes it's enough just to privately forgive.

Treat yourself to a professional pedicure.

Go with a friend to a nearby amusement park or carnival. Hop on a merry-go-round. Play the carny games. Try the roller coaster. Ride the Ferris wheel. Steer a bumper car. Eat some fried dough. And look at the expressions on the faces of your fellow fun-loving fairgoers.

Spend a half an hour just stretching
every muscle in your body.

Go to your hairdresser and ask for a whole new
look—new cut, new style, new color, new you!

Go out and buy something new for your house.
It might be just a little knickknack.

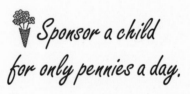

Sponsor a child
for only pennies a day.

Take a drive when the leaves are changing color—
not to *go* anywhere, but just to observe nature's glory.

*Leave the ham sandwich, bowl of soup, or tuna salad for
another day and go someplace exotic for lunch.*

When you wake up, listen to your favorite music for ten minutes—not the morning radio or TV weather you're used to tuning in when you first wake up. (If you share your bed with someone who gets up later than you, earphones will keep you from disturbing your partner's slumber.) Take your music into the bathroom with you as you brush your teeth, wash your face, and so forth.

❦

Tell a child about your favorite memory of childhood.
Relive it happily and tell it in such a way
that the child gets caught up in it, too.

Perfumed Bath

Did someone give you a holiday or birthday gift of a perfume that's not exactly your style? Here's a great way to use it without wearing a scent you're not happy with: Take a perfumed bath. Be profligate. Be extravagant. Really pour the perfume into the water. Turn the tap on as warm as you can take it, start filling the tub, and as the water pours in, add the perfume to the stream of running water. Remain in the bathroom as the tub fills, inhaling the intoxicating, decadent, strong scent. Illuminate the bathroom with candles and turn off the electric lights. Step into the tub, ease into the water, stretch out, lie back, and luxuriate.

Adopt a four-legged best friend, or buy an exotic pet.
Or, just visit a pet shop and enjoy looking around,
even if you don't bring someone home with you.

ℬ

Sleep in and have someone special
deliver you breakfast in bed.

✥

Apply to be on a reality television series
or game show.

✥

Purchase stock in your favorite company.

Take yourself on a date
to the top of a mountain.
Bring your camera or your sketch pad.

Take photos of subjects that represent things
or experiences you would like to have.
Create a collage of the photos and imagine
these things are now a part of your life.

Read a biography of someone you admire.

Even if you're not a classical music enthusiast, listen
to a good recording of Tchaikovsky's violin concerto.

Go to a sidewalk café with a good friend or alone, enjoy a cup of coffee, a glass of wine, or a bite of food, and people-watch as you eat or sip.

Just as there are comfort foods, there are also comfort materials. Do you have a favorite bathrobe, favorite sweater, or other garment you like to put on when you need warmth, comfort, and/or reassurance? The next time you want to be good to yourself, why not start by putting on your best comfort clothing—even if it's summer and your favorite comfort clothing is a warm, fuzzy robe!

Put some money
in your savings account.
(If you don't have one,
start one.)

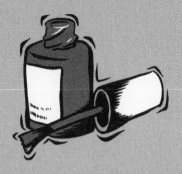

Polish your fingernails or toenails in a really offbeat, decorative way—two-tone polish, or polish laced with glitter, or polish with a small fake "jewel" centered on every nail, or alternating colors of polish from toe to toe. Or, get long acrylic fingernails.

Order some extravagant personalized stationery
for yourself—perhaps even with raised lettering.
It could be on parchment, linen, vellum,
or whatever attracts you.

Experiment in front of the mirror—
with your makeup, your hair, or (preferably)
both—and give yourself a whole new look.

Put on a funky hat, tie it on with a long, silk scarf,
and go for a drive with all the windows rolled down.

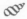

Buy a new workout outfit—you may
be inspired to hit the treadmill or the trail!

Learn to throw pottery, or paint some ready-to-be-finished pieces.

Get your car repainted in a "different" color, one that proclaims it uniquely yours. (Robin's egg blue? Shocking pink? Cheery yellow? Mint green?) (My last car was lilac!) Not only will your car get attention (of the good sort), but it will be less desirable to steal (more easily identified) and easier to find in parking lots, too.

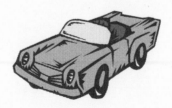

Walk around a craft store, investigating possible new hobbies. You can learn to make soap, or bread, or model planes or boats, or create and arrange silk flowers. You may find a wonderful new interest!

Visit a planetarium or an observatory.

Design a greeting card you would like to receive.

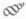

If you like to shop, go visit a different mall than the one you're accustomed to going to, or to a strip shopping center you've never investigated. Check out the stores, the merchandise, the displays.

Cheer someone else up.
Sometimes looking at the problems
of others helps us put our own into
perspective——and even if that doesn't
happen, you'll feel better just for
having made someone else happier.

The next time you're a passenger on a boring car ride, look at the various vehicles you pass—cars, trucks, even bicycles—and imagine they're all animals. What animal does each vehicle remind you of?

Buy cheery office supplies—sticky notes in bright colors, fun pens, slick new folders.

Bake yourself a chocolate cake— and be sure to lick the bowl and beaters.

Write a poem—any subject. The meter doesn't have to be perfect. You don't have to ever show the poem to anyone. Just write it for your own pleasure.

Buy yourself an especially cute—or huge—stuffed animal. Name it. Tell it a story.

Go on a cruise.

Visit an upscale art gallery
even if you can't afford to do anything but look.

Get in your car and just go
for a drive—wherever the nose
of your car leads you!
Explore a road you've never taken,
a part of the city or the countryside
that you've never explored,
or even a part you think you
know very well but will try
to see today with new eyes.
Make as many discoveries as you can.

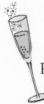

Have champagne with your breakfast.
Perch an orange slice on the rim of your glass.

Visit a store that sells luxurious merchandise and touch the fine things you see there, stroking or otherwise tactilely experiencing the store's goods. It might be a furniture store, clothing boutique, jewelry counter, antiques shop, or some other type of emporium. But don't just look—feel!

Buy yourself that piece of jewelry you've been admiring in that shop window for the last month, or some totally outrageous earrings. Tell yourself it's an early birthday or holiday present—from yourself—and ask to have the item gift wrapped.

Reserve a trip on a Mississippi paddleboat.

Run through the sprinklers
as if you were still a kid ...
and for just a few minutes,
you will be.

Turn off the phone and let
the machine pick up your calls.

Write your autobiography.

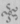

Buy a glamorous wig.

Get vanity plates for your car—with your name,
initials, nickname, or a word of your choice.

Visit a comedy club and laugh yourself silly.

Buy yourself a cheesecake.
(Call up your best friend and offer her half.)

Visit an elderly person and share stories all afternoon.

Decide what chore you least want to do—
the nagging problem around your home that's
been on your mind for weeks or months now,
but you keep putting it off—and do it.
Doing the chore may not feel like being good
to yourself, but oh!, will you feel good when
you know it's not hanging over you anymore.

*Visit a friend who grows houseplants
and come home with a handful of cuttings
you can root and grow at your house.*

Buy yourself a toy or game from a toy store.
It could be a Frisbee, an adult board game,
or something else intended for grown-ups,
but it might also be a kids' toy. Get it—just as long
as it's something *you'll* enjoy playing with!

Take some bread to the nearest pond or lake,
and see if you can get the ducks to eat from your hand.

Go for a swim. If it isn't summer, perhaps there's a
nearby indoor pool at a hotel, gym, Y, or even
a school that's open to the public for a price,
if only at certain hours. If you have your own pool,
sneak out after the kids are asleep and indulge
in some wickedly luxurious skinny-dipping
or float on an air raft (weather permitting!).

Concoct an outrageous "Dagwood" sandwich.

Lighten Up with Candles

On a gray day, a lonely evening, or any time your life seems too blah or the world seems too dull, light candles throughout the house. Subdue (or totally turn off) the electric lights, so they don't compete with the candles' warm glow. Now you have a choice: You can do the sewing you were going to do, the work you'd brought home from the office, or whatever had been on your agenda; or you can write a poem, inspired by the candle glow; or you can just sit and reflect (or simply daydream). (Hint: Classical music, particularly violin music, makes the best background for candlelight.)

Buy a new pair of glamorous glasses
(or sunglasses) with strikingly different
frames from the ones you wear now.

Go outside with a child or your special someone
and two water pistols. Ready? Aim. Fire!

Cheer your team at a live sporting event!
If there are no professional teams nearby,
why not go to your local high school?
Getting caught up in team spirit
will definitely boost your spirit!

Learn how to be a ventriloquist.

Buy a coffee-table or guide book about
an exotic location you've always dreamed of.

Go to a restaurant that serves a cuisine you've never
tried before, whether Vietnamese, Hungarian,
Turkish, or Tex-Mex. Experiment. Be daring.

Plan an afternoon around
preparing to watch the sun set.

Learn to quilt, knit, crochet, or do needlepoint.

Go to a museum you've never visited—
preferably something offbeat.

Call or go online and request a catalog from
the local college or the local high school's
community education (adult education) department.

Have chocolate for breakfast.

Got an old favorite dress, blouse, or pair of pants
that you never wear anymore because it's too
tight/loose/shabby/out of style?
Take it to the tailor and let him or her do something
about letting it out, taking it in, refurbishing it, or
otherwise making it wearable again.

Buy yourself an expensive pen—
maybe even an old-fashioned fountain pen.

*Do something particularly
nice for someone else.
You'll feel good too.*

Throw a big, fluffy towel in the dryer. While it heats up in there, run a bath. Remove the towel just before you get into the tub. When you get out, the towel will still be nice and hot.

Get a professional makeover.

Visit open houses, even if you have no intention of buying. It's fun to see how other people live, and you might get some great ideas about your own home.

Get together with a group of friends—male, female, young, older—and just sit back and yak. This could be a bull session, a joke-fest, or a brainstorming session on "How we could improve our lives." It could even be a "What's wrong with the world and how I'd fix it if I were in charge" session. Or a gripe session in which you all air your grievances (not with each other). You might be surprised at what you learn—someone may actually have a constructive suggestion on what to do about what's bugging you.

Enjoy the Beach Twelve Months a Year

Walk on the beach, even if it isn't summer and "beach weather." A windswept autumn beach, snow-sheened wonderland, or breeze-kissed springtime sand-strip can be a great place to get in touch with your thoughts and dreams. Hunt for seashells on the beach. Look for a variety of types, each in perfect condition, or concentrate on one less-common type (think starfish, conch, or sand dollar, rather than clam or mussel). Display them on a shelf, on your coffee table, on your dresser, or on your mirrored perfume tray.

Call up your mom or dad (or another relative
you spent a lot of time with in your childhood—
a sibling, grandparent, favorite aunt or uncle,
or cousin) and reminisce about your childhood.
Ask your relative to tell you stories of "the
old days" that you may have forgotten.

Pose for a glamour portrait.

Buy yourself a music box, one that looks attractive
and plays a tune you like. (You might even
decide to start a whole collection.)

Go to a church, synagogue, or mosque. You don't have to be a member of the congregation. And you can choose to go during a worship service or at a time when you're likely to have the sanctuary to yourself. Even if you're not particularly religious, the beauty and peace of the surroundings should speak to your soul and renew you.

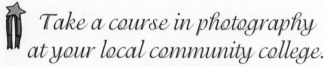

Take a course in photography at your local community college.

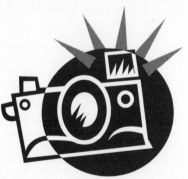

Remember the relay races you ran as a child, in which all the members of each team were required to duck-walk, frog-hop, crab-walk, hop on one leg, skip, or move themselves in other unusual ways from Point A to Point B? Get together with one or more friends and try to replicate all those odd gaits now. Can you crab-walk across your family room, skip down the hallway, duck-walk across your backyard? Award prizes for winners.

Hint to someone special that you'd like the services
of a "personal chef" who'll come to your house
for your next birthday and cook a splendid feast
for you and your family and/or guests.

Teach yourself a magic trick.

Plant flowers in your yard in a pattern
the shape of a heart—or perhaps patterned
so that they form your initials.

An Attitude of Gratitude

Write a note to someone who has made a difference in your life—whether recently or in the distant past. It could be a boss, an employee, a co-worker, a teacher, a relative, a friend, a neighbor, or anyone else. Tell them *how* they made a difference, why they were so important to you, and how much you appreciate what they did for you/taught you/showed you. We often don't know when we've left footprints on someone's life or heart. You'll not only make their day when they receive the note, *you'll* feel a glow for writing it. If the person you're thanking has passed on, place the letter at their gravesite, or send it to their next of kin.

Treat yourself to a facial.

If you usually shop bargain racks, discount chains,
or off-price stores, buy yourself one *good* dress,
pantsuit, or set of coordinates—something
that firmly announces "quality" to all who see it.

Buy yourself a CD burner and copy all those
great LPs you haven't listened to in years!

If you're single, go on a blind date.

Explore a part of your town—
a park, a neighborhood,
a playground—
you're not familiar with.
Make it an all-day outing.
Pretend you're a tourist.
Bring your camera!

Buy a few less-common herbs and spices
and experiment with them in your cooking.
If you substitute or add exotic or simply different
herbs/spices, you'll give new life to a possibly tired
old favorite such as meat loaf or baked chicken.

Share one of your favorite websites with a friend
who would really enjoy visiting it. Ask the friend
to send you a link to a really super site in return.

Boil a pot of water and drop in some
simmering potpourri (or vanilla essence).
Scent the whole house, or a large part of it.
Take deep breaths.
Enjoy.

Hire someone to come in and clean your carpets.

Do something you thought you were too old
and serious for—surfing, windsurfing,
jet-skiing, skydiving, white-water rafting,
or even just dancing till dawn.

Have "breakfast" for dinner
one night, just because.
Fix eggs, bacon, waffles,
or oatmeal—or all of them!
Whatever your idea is of a
satisfying, tummy-warming
breakfast. Go ahead—pour a
big bowl of sugary kid cereal,
if that's what you enjoy!

In winter's cold and early dark, try on a
bathing suit or sun dress and remember
that summer is only half a year (or less) away.

Buy a bubble wand and bubble solution.
Go outdoors and have fun with it.
(Bringing a child along is fine but not necessary.)

Bake your favorite cookies—
and save some of the dough to nibble.

Buy your own star through a star registry
and name it after yourself.

Host a White Elephant Exchange

Got a dress you no longer like, a good pair of shoes that never fit right, a serving dish your great-aunt sent you that isn't quite your taste (and isn't returnable)? How about a scarf you never wear, a bottle of perfume you don't care for, or books you've read and don't want to keep? Host a party, asking each guest to bring similar items from their homes. Spread them out and watch your friends grab them up—and see what treasures you can grab for yourself.

Start a memory book. Get yourself a notebook and a pen that slides along the paper. Begin to make a record of your best memories. It can be best memories about grade school, high school, college, when the kids were little. It can be long-ago. It can be just yesterday. Make a record of what you like to remember. It will help you remember what's important to you. It will cheer you up when you're feeling down.

Buy a new pillow that's just the right degree of firmness to suit you. Sweet dreams!

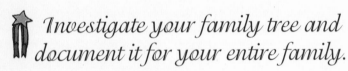 *Investigate your family tree and document it for your entire family.*

Stretch out on the couch with your favorite music on the stereo. You probably play this album—whether it's Beethoven or the Beatles, Madonna or Mariah, Gershwin or gospel—often as you go about your days; it's background music to make your tasks easier. But when's the last time you really *listened* to it—just stretched out and really paid attention?

Go get a psychic reading—
even if you think it's pure hogwash,
in which case it'll be good for a laugh,
or for the fun of proving how wrong
the psychic reader was.

Change your sheets, even though you just changed
them two or three days ago and it's not time again yet.
You'll enjoy the feel of the fresh, crisp, cool linen
when you go to bed tonight.

Have one of the rooms in your
house repainted, or do it yourself.
If you have four off-white walls,
consider painting one of them
in a contrasting color.

Hop on a bus.
Observe your fellow passengers—
it's fun to people-watch
or get to know the passing scenery.

Color all the pictures in a coloring book.

Visit a chiropractor and have your back realigned,
even if you don't need it.

L ie on your back in the backyard and look at the clouds. Or just stand and look up. Remember when you were a kid, and the clouds all looked like lions, castles, or ponies? What do these clouds look like to you now? If you want, make up stories about them, too, the way you did when you were younger.

Create a rock garden.

People-Watch with Imagination

Go somewhere where there are many people—a busy city street, a train terminal, a department store— and, as you look at your fellow humans, devise back-stories for many of them. *Who is this woman? Where is she from? What's her name? Why is she here today? What does she do for a living—or, if she doesn't work, who supports her, and how does she spend her days? What does she most want out of life?* Of course you don't *know* the facts— mostly, you'll make them up, but you *can* rely on visual clues to help you. Is her clothing neat or bedraggled, stylish or timeless or passé, well-fitting or perhaps a hand-me-down? How much makeup does she wear? What does her hair look like? What is she carrying? Is she suntanned, wrinkled, weary-looking? Is she carrying anything?

Buy a large bag of your favorite candy—
and eat until you're full.

Recreate a food you remember from your childhood and haven't eaten since. It could be something your mom fixed for you regularly (or as an occasional treat), a snack you were fond of fixing for yourself after school, or your favorite ice cream sundae. Whatever that treat is—blueberry pancakes, a peanut butter and banana sandwich (with marshmallow fluff?), or a butterscotch sundae with maple walnut ice cream and an extra cherry—indulge yourself.

Call up your best friend and agree to trade presents
this week, even though it isn't your birthday or hers,
Christmas, Chanukah, or any other holiday.
Shop for the perfect gift for her, and have fun
guessing what she is giving you in return.

Buy new drapes or curtains for all your windows
and surprise yourself with how new your house looks!

Take a train ride to the next state.

If you don't own a bicycle, borrow or rent one
and go for a ride. Choose whether to explore
nearby areas, take a longish ride to a less-familiar
place, or explore an area far from your home.

Go for a walk in the rain.

Join whatever self-help group or organization
best suits your purposes, from Weight-Watchers
to Al-Anon, from a single-parent help group
to a Bible discussion group. You're likely to meet
one or more new friends—and become
a better friend to yourself, too.

*Make yourself a few sachets (or buy some)
and tuck them into various drawers and even closets
(certainly the linen closet, for one!) around the house.*

Buy a new set of sheets, a new bedspread,
or a thick comforter in an outrageous color
or a gorgeous pattern. Or buy some satin
sheets and matching decorative pillows.

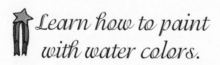 *Learn how to paint with water colors.*

Has it just snowed? Be a kid again—in a new way. Fill a turkey baster—or even better, a water pistol—with a solution of water and food coloring. Paint your name, some hearts, and other pictures in the snow.

Join a community theatre.

Buy some oranges and treat yourself to some fresh-squeezed juice. The stuff you usually buy in cartons—or frozen concentrate—may be acceptable for your average hurried morning, but real fresh orange juice is much more of a treat.

Look over your things-to-do list, choose all the easiest/quickest items on it and put an asterisk next to them. Do them, crossing each item off as it's accomplished. After you've finished, or at a point when it's getting late and you need to stop, look at your list and feel a swell of satisfaction as you see how many items you've crossed off.

Alone when you'd rather not be? And you have no plans with any of your friends? Drop in on a neighbor. (You may want to call first, if you're not sure the timing's good.) It's nice to reinforce our relationships with those who live around us.

Read and then recycle that pile of magazines
that's been sitting there for months.
Catch up on your reading *and* make
a pile of clutter disappear from the house!

Run barefoot
through tall grass.

Rent a ride in a hot air balloon.

Invite a friend over to play games, whether it's a
boxed game, a card game, or a game such as charades
that needs no special equipment at all.

Treat yourself to a professional massage. Or trade
massages with a friend. Have a nice heart-to-heart talk
while you massage each other. Or do it in total
silence and let each of you lose herself in thought.

Install dimmer switches to control at least
one lamp or the ceiling fixture in your
living room and bedroom.

Meander Down Memory Lane

Take a trip to your childhood hometown and revisit all the old places you remember. Ring the doorbell of your old home, explain to the present residents that you used to live there, and ask them if you might come in and look around for old time's sake. Notice the changes in the building and property, for better and for worse, as well as simply different. Remember the special memories associated with that house, and glow as you remember them. Now remember the bad times, and reflect on how much better your life is now in those regards.

Lie down on a shaggy or soft-and-furry rug
and roll around—preferably without any clothes on.

Call up your friends and have a spontaneous,
come-as-you-are party. Everyone must attend
in exactly what they were wearing when you
called—unless a person was in the shower at the
time, in which case a robe will be allowed.

Weave a chain of daisies or even dandelions to hang
in your office or bedroom, or to wear as a bracelet.

Go to a driving range and hit a bucket of golf balls.

Plan a family reunion.

Use different spices on your popcorn—
garlic, celery salt, paprika—experiment!

Set up a birdfeeder outside your bedroom window.

Sew sequins on that tired-looking old blouse
or sweater and give it a new life.

Do nothing!
Give yourself permission
to do absolutely nothing.
Lounge, daydream, sip coffee,
and just slouch around.
If you must do *something*,
make sure it's a lovely waste
of time, not something
legitimately productive.

If you find it cathartic, organize your dresser and your bathroom cabinets. If you think the prospect of organizing those places will stress you out even more, by all means, shut the doors and go have an iced tea!

Throw a costume ball!

Paint or stick glow-in-the-dark stars on your bedroom ceiling (and perhaps on your living room ceiling as well).

Get a foot massage.

Lightly spray your sheets with perfume just before bedtime.

Dust off your roller skates, inline skates,
or ice skates, and go for a spin on the nearest rink
or just up and down your sidewalk.

Go fabric shopping and have that worn or dirty
chair reupholstered in a fabric you just love, one
that gives a whole new look to your living room.
Or, if you can't afford reupholstering,
buy new slipcovers for a fraction of the cost!

Go to a nightclub where there's dancing, and bring a
partner, even if he's just a good friend, so you can be
sure of getting in plenty of time on the dance floor.

Have a snowball fight with your kids,
special someone, or best friend.

Check your closets, drawers, attic,
garage, or basement to see what
you can post on an online auction.
The sale of those clothes that no longer
fit may finance a clothes-shopping spree.
The sale of the coin collection or butterfly
collection you're no longer interested in
may finance your next hobby.
Or the sale of the baseball cards your dad
left you or the old desk from Aunt Edna
may finance your child's first year
in college or that Mediterranean cruise
you've always wanted to take!

Buy a special painting, poster, mask, scroll,
or other artwork for a wall in your house.

Shoot a roll or two of photos of your family.
Go to a one-hour developer
and enjoy the pictures tonight.

Bookworm-for-a-Day

Spend the day luxuriating with books. Go through your bookshelves. Cull the books you no longer want and donate them to your local library (or an abused women's shelter, or any worthy cause that has a thrift shop). Select a few old favorites you haven't read in a long while and put them aside on your night table and get ready for visits with a few good old friends. Go to the bookstore and buy your favorite author's new book in hardcover, especially if you've always waited for paperback. Then, go to a used book store and stock up on goodies. Afterwards, stop by the library and borrow an armload of books—not books that you need for your college course, not books that your child needs for school, not books that you need to use for research for the office or for your next writing project—books you're borrowing just for fun! Tonight, curl up in bed with all your newfound (or rediscovered) books and pore over them while sipping wine and listening to your favorite music. Doesn't that sound like a heavenly day?

Apply your favorite body lotion from your nose to your toes.

Hire a magician to entertain the guests at your next dinner party or cocktail party. Your friends will praise you, and you'll have a wonderful time yourself. (How often are your parties really fun for *you* rather than being more like work?)

Eat a meal—breakfast, lunch, dinner, your choice—in
your backyard (when the weather suits), eating under
the trees or near fragrant bushes or in any place where
you're enjoying both the meal and the outdoors.
(If it's dinner, and it's not midsummer, when dark
comes late, you can dine under the stars.)

Do an informational interview with someone
whose career has always interested you.
Or visit a local college and ask how they
can help you make your life more fulfilling.

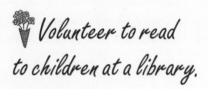 *Volunteer to read to children at a library.*

Go to a crafts store and buy the necessary supplies for making earrings. Some crafts stores also sell instruction books for this craft (and others); if your local crafts store doesn't, your bookstore surely does. Learn to make pretty and/or exotic earrings of beads, shells, feathers, and imitation gems.

Cine-magic

Rent your all-time favorite movie. Or, rent a three-hanky special at the video store, curl up with a glass of wine and a box of tissues, and let yourself have a good cathartic cry. Or, rent your favorite movie from childhood (no, the people at the video store really aren't staring at you). Enjoy the magic of great cinematic storytelling.

Throw yourself and your friends a pizza party—
use a variety of exotic toppings, such as pineapple,
sage, gorgonzola cheese, and walnuts, to start!

Plan to visit the studio audience
of your favorite television show.
Write, call, or go online for tickets,
which are usually free!

Create your own list of little indulgences
and treat yourself to every one of them!

Be good to yourself.